HSE

614.8

Managing skin exposure risks at work

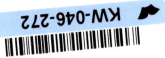

HSE Books

© Crown copyright 2009

First published 2009

ISBN 978 0 7176 6309 5

This guidance is issued by the Health and Safety Executive. Following the guidance is not compulsory and you are free to take other action. But if you do follow the guidance you will normally be doing enough to comply with the law. Health and safety inspectors seek to secure compliance with the law and may refer to this guidance as illustrating good practice.

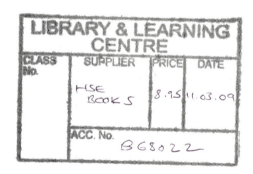

Contents

Introduction

Is this guidance useful to me?

1   Many materials used at work can affect the skin or can pass through the skin and cause diseases elsewhere in the body. If you are an employer, health and safety adviser, trainer or safety representative you can help prevent these disabling diseases. This guidance will help you with practical advice. It covers:

- the protective role of the skin;
- ill health arising from skin exposure;
- recognising potential skin exposure in your workplace;
- managing skin exposure to prevent disease.

What does health and safety law say about this?

2   Many employers are unaware that they have legal duties to assess the health risks from skin exposure to hazardous substances at work. They must prevent or, where this is not reasonably practicable, adequately control exposure to the hazards by using and maintaining suitable controls. This book can help employers comply with their legal duties. There is more information on the law in Appendix 1.

A cross section of the outer layer of skin cells to illustrate the potential pathways through which chemical absorption can take place. Chemicals can also enter the body through the openings in skin surface (eg around hair follicles and through the ducts of the sweat glands).

Why is the skin important?

3   The skin is the largest organ in the human body. Its main functions are to:

- provide a protective barrier against harmful substances;
- protect against injury;
- restrict the loss of moisture;
- reduce the harmful effects of UV radiation;
- act as a sensory organ (eg touch, temperature);
- help regulate body temperature;
- help detect and protect against infections;
- produce vitamin D.

4   The skin is made up of two main layers, the epidermis and dermis. The outer layer, the epidermis, provides the skin's barrier function. However, it is not a perfect barrier – it limits the amount of material that can pass through it to affect other parts of the body.

5   If the moisture content of the epidermis is too high or too low, it can affect the skin's barrier properties. If it is too dry, for example when working in a low-humidity room, the skin dehydrates, becomes rough, thickened and flaky and can crack through loss of elasticity. If it is too moist, for example due to prolonged contact with water, the skin becomes over-hydrated, impairing its barrier function.

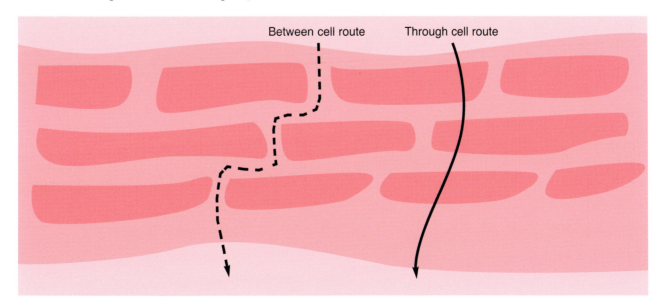

Between cell route   Through cell route

What health problems can occur through skin contact?

6   Some substances can pass though the skin and cause diseases in other parts of the body. Other substances can cause 'local effects', which are limited to the skin itself. Dealing with local effects first, there are four main groups of substances that can cause skin problems, mostly at the site of skin contact:

- corrosive substances that can lead to burns;
- irritant substances that can lead to irritant contact dermatitis;
- sensitising substances that can lead to allergic contact dermatitis;
- substances that cause other diseases, eg urticaria, acne, skin cancer.

Burns

7   Severe skin damage (burns) can follow brief skin contact with a corrosive substance, eg wet cement, strong acids and alkalis. This may lead to the skin scarring.

Irritant contact dermatitis (ICD)

8   Irritant contact dermatitis is a skin reaction leading to inflammation at the site of contact. Dry, red and itchy skin is a common first sign. Swelling, flaking, blistering, cracking and pain may follow. Usually, the inflammation subsides once the skin has healed. However, repeated contact may lead to 'hyper-irritability' – the skin becomes inflamed more readily than normal.

9   ICD can develop after regular contact with mild irritants such as detergents, weak acids or alkalis and some solvents. It can develop through 'wet work'. Wet work is the term used to describe prolonged or frequent contact with water (particularly in combination with soaps, cleaners and other chemicals). Wet work can cause the skin to over-hydrate. It is a leading cause of ICD but often goes unrecognised.

Allergic contact dermatitis (ACD)

10   Allergic contact dermatitis (or skin sensitisation) is an 'immunological response' to a sensitising substance (allergen). The signs and symptoms are difficult to distinguish from ICD. Sensitisation can develop over time and it may be weeks, months or even years before it becomes apparent. However, once a person has developed an allergy (is 'sensitised'), tiny amounts of the allergen will trigger ACD. By then, the only remedy is to prevent further exposure.

Other skin diseases

11   Urticaria is a skin condition that typically shows as a wheal (swelling) and flare (red mark) reaction. Skin irritants or allergens may cause it. It is different from ICD and ACD in that it quickly follows skin contact and disappears again within hours.

12   Skin cancer is one of the most common types of cancer. Signs of skin cancer may include a scaly patch of hard skin, a red lump or spot, an ulcer, a new mole, or a patch of skin that bleeds, oozes or has a crust. Polycyclic aromatic hydrogen compounds can cause skin cancer. Don't forget that skin cancer is a particular problem for outdoor workers exposed to ultraviolet rays from the skin.

13   Acne is an inflammatory disease of the sebaceous glands and hair follicles in the skin. Pimples and pustules (white-centred bumps) mark it. Grease and oils can cause 'oil acne' in mechanics and roofers can develop acne from exposure to pitch.

Systemic diseases following uptake through the skin

14   Many substances can pass through the skin and cause diseases in other parts of the body (systemic diseases). Examples include bladder and scrotal cancers, diseases of the kidneys, heart, circulatory and nervous systems, and poisoning. Some health effects can appear quickly, some can take months or years to appear (eg cancers). Whether or not a substance causes systemic disease by skin uptake, it is good practice to control skin exposure.

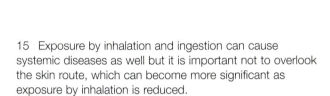

15 Exposure by inhalation and ingestion can cause systemic diseases as well but it is important not to overlook the skin route, which can become more significant as exposure by inhalation is reduced.

Case studies: Exposure to chemicals

When a worker in France was disposing of some industrial waste, he splattered 2,4 dichlorophenol over parts of his arm and thigh. This was on less than 10% of his body surface. He experienced a seizure within 20 minutes and died. (Kintz et al 1992)[1]

Two workers in a textile factory developed a brain disorder, primarily from skin exposure to ethylene glycol monomethyl ether. The poisoning happened when they used it as a cleaning agent, substituting it for acetone, which was unavailable due to a temporary shortage. (Ohi and Wegman 1978)[2]

What are the consequences of diseases?

16 For individual employees there is pain and suffering, with their social life affected. Some may have to give up their jobs. For employers, there are cost consequences such as sickness absence, loss of productivity and the potential for a criminal record. For society, there are costs such as disability living allowance, incapacity benefit and NHS resources for care or rehabilitation.

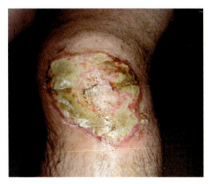

Cement burns to a construction worker's knee. This serious injury could have been prevented either by avoiding the need to kneel down in wet cement or by providing a suitable pair of knee protectors.

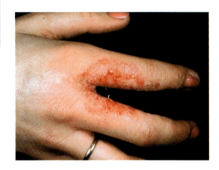

This hand shows irritant contact dermatitis. It is swollen, painful and infected.

How do I recognise a skin hazard?

17 Hazardous substances include:

- substances/products used directly in work activities (eg adhesives, paints, cleaning products);
- substances generated during work activities (eg rosin fumes from soldering, metal fumes from welding, wood dust from sanding);
- naturally occurring substances (eg grain dust, flour);
- biological agents (eg bacteria).

18 The first step in recognising a skin hazard is to identify substances either used or generated in your workplace. Next, decide which might cause health effects following skin exposure. There are information sources that help with these steps:

- HSE's 'Skin at work' web pages (www.hse.gov.uk/skin);
- substances with a 'skin notation' (symbol Sk) in *EH40/2005 Workplace exposure limits*;[3]
- the product label – look for the risk and safety phrases in Table 1;
- trade associations, trade journals or trade websites.

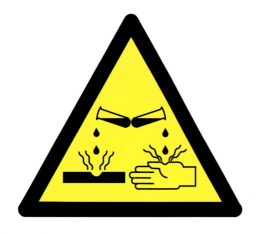

Chemicals marked with this symbol are corrosive, they may destroy living tissue on contact.

Risk phrase – effects on the skin	
R21	Harmful in contact with the skin
R24	Toxic in contact with the skin
R34	Causes burns
R35	Causes severe burns
R38	Irritating to the skin
R43	May cause sensitisation by skin contact
R66	Repeated exposure may cause skin dryness or cracking

Risk phrase – uptake through the skin	
R21	Harmful in contact with the skin (and combinations, eg R20/21/22)
R24	Toxic in contact with the skin (and combinations, eg R48/24)
R27	Very toxic in contact with the skin (and combinations, eg R39/27)

Safety phrases	
S24	Avoid contact with skin
S25	Avoid contact with eyes
S26	In case of contact with eyes, rinse immediately with plenty of water and seek medical advice
S27	Take off all contaminated clothing immediately
S28	After contact with skin, wash immediately with plenty of ... (as specified by the manufacturer)
S36	Wear suitable protective clothing
S37	Wear suitable gloves
S39	Wear suitable eye and face protection

Table 1 Risk and safety phrases
These are applied to 'classify' products that cause effects following skin exposure. The CHIP Regulations[4] require chemical suppliers to identify the hazards (or dangers) of the chemicals they supply.

How do I assess the risks?

19   The 'risk' is the likelihood that workers' skin will come into contact with hazardous substances that could affect their health. 'Assessment' means deciding who might be harmed and how:

■   Do you have to use the substance and, if so, how much is used?
■   How often is it used, and by how many workers?
■   How is the substance handled – can you handle it in a way to avoid skin contact?
■   Which parts of the skin are exposed and for how long?

20   Remember those cleaners, visitors, contractors and maintenance workers etc who may not be in the workplace all the time.

21   You can often do the assessment by simply watching the tasks. Where cases of skin exposure are less predictable or less obvious, using colour-indicating wipes or pads can help you detect skin or surface contamination (your trade association may be able to help you find a supplier). For situations that are more complex or where very toxic materials are used, you are advised to seek the help of a health and safety professional such as an occupational hygienist. They will help you to assess the risks and will advise you on the appropriate methods to manage those risks to prevent ill health.

Exposure pathways

22   An 'exposure pathway' is the link between a hazard source and a worker. Skin exposure can occur by several pathways:

■   immersion – the skin is submerged into a liquid or powder;
■   splashes – from decanting or mixing of liquids and powders;
■   deposition – when droplets, dusts, fumes or aerosols contact the skin, either as part of a work activity or incidental to it (eg emission from a nearby process);
■   contact with contaminated surfaces. This can happen in a variety of ways:
    -    directly handling a contaminated workpiece;
    -    contact with contaminated work surfaces;
    -    residues on hands transferred to the eyes, nose and mouth;
    -    residues on hands transferred to tools, paperwork and food;
    -    removing contaminated PPE incorrectly.

Case study: Cement dust

Tim's four-year-old daughter got a painful rash that would not go away. Tim took her to several doctors, but the ointments they applied did not make a difference. Then Tim listened to a toolbox talk on preventing dermatitis at work. Tim works on a building site using cement. He realised his daughter may have been exposed to cement dust.

Tim began following the precautions mentioned in the talk. He cleaned the inside of his car and now always removes his work overalls before getting into it. He also follows the guidance on washing and caring for his skin. Within a few weeks his daughter's problem was gone – Tim's skin is better too.

The risks from wet work

23   There is no hard and fast rule on when wet work is likely to be a risk. However, as a rule of thumb, prolonged contact of more than about 2 hours, or more than 20-40 hand washes/contacts a day, are likely to lead to dermatitis. Dermatitis from wet work is common in trades such as hairdressing, metal machining, catering, cleaning and healthcare.

Case study: Repeated hand washing

Fifty-five employees working for a meat-processing company were suffering from hand dermatitis. Repeated hand washing with a cleanser was routine (30-40 washes a day). Hands were often immersed in 'over-hot', softened, water dosed with chlorine dioxide. Gloves were not routinely used. No skin care regime was in place. No skin checking was carried out, so early warnings of a problem were missed.

When the outbreak happened, the company sought the help of a consultant, who sorted the problem. His advice was to:

■   reduce water temperature and control it at 32° C;
■   regulate chlorine dioxide dosing at a continuous, ideal level;
■   reduce washing by 30% throughout a shift (this still maintained adequate food hygiene standards);
■   supply and encourage the use of appropriate moisturising cream;
■   introduce skin checking.

How can I manage risks to prevent ill health?

24   Prevention is always better than cure. If you identify a skin contamination problem, you need to develop measures to adequately control the risk. This will reduce the likelihood of health effects occurring.

25   Managing work to prevent ill health from skin exposure can be summed up in three key steps: avoid; protect; check.

- Avoid or reduce contact with materials that cause skin/systemic problems.
- Protect the skin.
- Check for early signs of disease.

Case study: Engineering controls can reduce contact

Sam was a spray painter working in a furniture factory. He sprayed furniture on an overhead conveyor belt wearing a respirator. He stood between the furniture and the exhaust vent at the rear of the area when spraying the back of each piece. He occasionally wore rubber gloves, but they weren't always available.

When a new paint was introduced, Sam developed a rash on his arms. Within a week or so this had spread to his legs and neck. Shortly after that, Sam began to develop breathing difficulties. The new paint was epoxy-based, this can cause allergies. Sam had developed allergic contact dermatitis and asthma; he eventually had to give up work. This could have been prevented if the right precautions had been used.

- Epoxy-based paints should only be sprayed in an enclosed booth or room.
- Sprayers should be provided with air-fed respiratory protection.
- Sprayers should be provided with suitable personal protective equipment.
- Good washing facilities and skin creams should be provided.
- Health surveillance should be carried out.

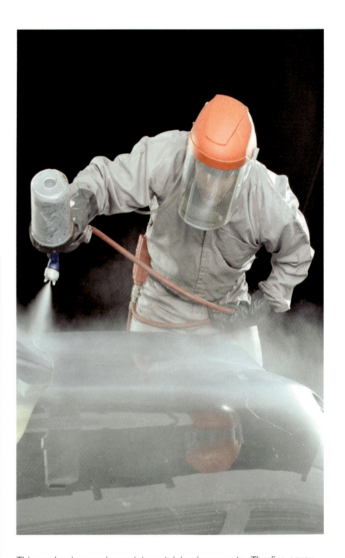

This worker is spraying paint containing isocyanate. The fine spray, not normally seen with the naked eye, is shown up with the use of 'Tyndall illumination'. Skin and inhalation exposure to isocyanates has the potential to cause skin allergies and asthma. It is crucial that the right controls are used.

How should I avoid or reduce contact with harmful materials?

Avoid contact by elimination

26   This is most feasible at the 'process design' stage. For existing systems, 'elimination' usually means a change of process, for example removing paint by scraping instead of using solvents. However, if this introduces other risks, such as noise, dust or musculoskeletal problems, these must be controlled too.

Avoid contact by substitution

27   If elimination is not possible, you should substitute or replace the substance with something less harmful. For example, use less concentrated products, replace solvent-based products with water-based ones and replace surfactant degreasers with milder products.

28   Substituting the physical form of a substance may also reduce the potential for skin contact. Use granulated or liquid formulations rather than powders to reduce the spread of dust. Use pre-packaged forms of a substance to avoid contact during scooping or weighing.

Avoid or reduce contact by using engineering controls

29   'Engineering controls' include containment (eg a glove box or closed reactor) and partial enclosure with some form of local exhaust ventilation (LEV).

30   Engineering controls can be very effective in controlling skin contact during normal operations. However, there will be a potential for contact during cleaning, maintenance and repair operations. For such cases, controls might include procedures such as defined decontamination procedures and permits to work.

Avoid or reduce contact by using a 'safe working distance'

31   Sometimes, the work means having the skin (usually the hands) close to the hazardous substance. The next option is to put a 'safe working distance' (SWD) between the skin and the hazardous substance. The greater the distance between the worker and the source of contamination, the less likely it is that contact will occur.

32   Use automated handling systems rather than manual handling. Use tools and equipment (eg tongs, hooks, scoops) for handling work items rather than using the hands as tools. Where tools have handles, choose a long-handled tool over a short-handled one.

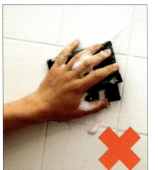 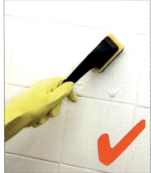

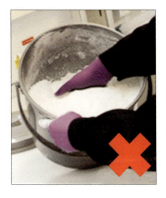 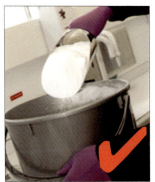

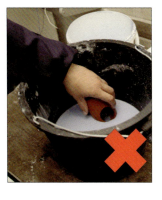 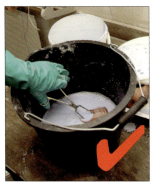

Distance your skin from chemicals and wet work.

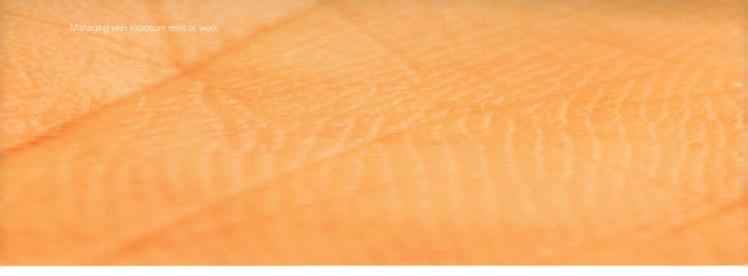

Case study: Handling solvent-soaked material

An inspector visited a factory producing coated fabrics. Workers handled solvent-soaked coating material, transferring lumps of it to a coating machine and then spreading it out with their hands. They did this for most of the day.

The inspector recognised that handling solvent-soaked material can cause irritant contact dermatitis and if the solvent passes through the skin it can cause ill health to other parts of the body. The inspector told them how to improve the situation.

- The material could be transferred using a semi-automated dispenser, operated by a compressed air plunger on demand by the operator.
- The spreading could be done using a suitable stainless-steel spatula, which would prevent the hands coming into contact with the material.
- Using the above procedures eliminates the need for cleaning the hands with solvents.

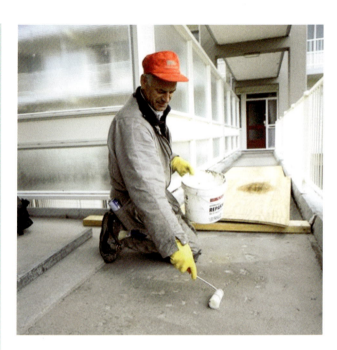

A floor coating being applied by a worker who is kneeling down and using a short-handled spreader.

Avoid or reduce contact by using procedural controls

33   Prevent or minimise access to areas where there is a risk of skin contact.

34   Put barriers between contaminated and clean work areas to prevent the spread of contamination.

35   Use spillage controls, eg using drip trays, to prevent the spread of contamination and make cleaning up spills easier.

36   When surface contamination is inevitable, reduce the impact by providing impermeable, easy-to-clean work surfaces. Clean them regularly. Alternatively, reduce contamination by using disposable, absorbent paper lining, with regular replacement.

37   Effective supervision will show you whether you are maintaining an adequate standard of control.

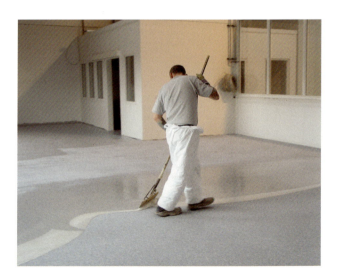

With the help of a long-handled spreader, an adequate safe working distance has been applied, reducing the likelihood of contact with the coating. It reduces the potential for back problems too.

(Photo courtesy of European Epoxy Project Team and IVAM, The Netherlands.)

What should I do to protect the skin?

Protect the skin by using personal protective equipment (PPE)

38   PPE is an important control option when other reasonably practicable methods of control do not give enough protection. However, it is important to remember that PPE has a number of limitations:

- it can only protect the wearer;
- it has to be the right material and the right size;
- it has to be put on, worn and taken off properly;
- it may limit the wearer's mobility or ability to communicate;
- its continued effectiveness will depend on proper cleaning, maintenance, training and supervision, to assure good control practice.

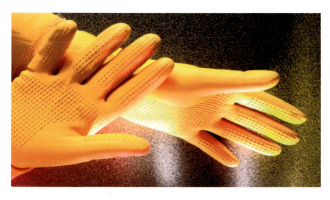

39   PPE is available in a wide range of natural and synthetic materials. Typical examples include gloves, aprons, overalls, footwear and respirators.

40   PPE needs to be 'fit for purpose' – the right quality and construction to give the protection needed. It should be 'CE marked', fit the wearer, be suitable for the task and compatible with any other PPE to be worn. Over-elaborate PPE can discourage its use.

41   Remember that PPE can increase the risk of skin exposure when used incorrectly. For example, contaminant trapped inside ill-fitting PPE can be held against unprotected skin.

42   Provide employees with information, instruction, training and adequate facilities for issue, use, cleaning, storage and maintenance of PPE. Employees need to follow the rules for PPE use, to wear it properly, look after it and report any loss, defects or other problems.

Case study: Benefits of PPE as part of a skin care regime

Joe was a part-time worker at a fast food restaurant. His duties were to fry food and clean down the equipment and stove at the end of the day.

Joe found that handling the moist foods and stove cleaners stung his hands and this, along with lots of hand washing, made his skin dry.

After seeing a doctor, Joe was told that he had irritant contact dermatitis, from wet work. Joe told his boss, who introduced some changes at work.

- A less hazardous cleaner is now used, which still does the job.
- Thick rubber gloves are used for cleaning.
- Vinyl food handler's gloves are used for handling moist foods.
- Workers use a moisturiser before breaks and at the end of shifts.
- Workers' skin is checked periodically.

Choosing and using protective gloves

43   Skin contact at work mostly occurs on the hands and forearms. There is a wide range of protective gloves on the market, the following guidance concerns choosing and using protective gloves to protect against hazardous substances and wet work only.

44   Take all the steps you can to avoid hand contact with substances before resorting to the use of protective gloves. If avoiding contact is impractical or gives insufficient protection, protective gloves are an appropriate solution.

45   The gloves you choose should be 'suitable' – they should match the work, the wearer and the work environment. There are five factors to consider:

- the substances handled;
- other hand hazards;
- the type and duration of contact;
- the wearer – in terms of size and comfort;
- the task and the need for robustness and sensitivity.

46   You can select protective gloves based on these criteria, but protective glove suppliers are best placed to help you with your selection. They will need information from you on the factors described in the previous paragraphs. To help with this, there is a memory aid sheet in Appendix 3; you can photocopy this, complete it and hand it to your supplier. You can also download copies from HSE's Skin at work web pages at www.hse.gov.uk/skin.

Substances handled

47   Gloves vary in design, material and thickness. No glove will protect against all substances and no glove will protect forever.

48   For 'wet work' choose a glove that meets the European Standard EN374-2. This shows that the gloves are waterproof.

49   To protect hands from substances/chemicals, choose a glove that meets the European Standard EN374-3, but be sure the glove material protects against the substances handled.

50   Glove manufacturers usually produce charts to show how well their gloves perform against a range of single substances/chemicals. The performance of glove materials can vary slightly from manufacturer to manufacturer, so check the right chart! These charts usually use three key terms: breakthrough time; permeation rate; and degradation.

- The time a chemical takes to work through (permeate) the glove material and reach the inside is the breakthrough time. The substances pass through the material without going through pinholes or pores or other visible openings. This is the maximum time that a glove remains effective. Choose a glove with a high breakthrough time.
- The permeation rate is the amount that then moves through. The higher the rate the more of the chemical will get through the glove. Choose a low permeation rate.
- Degradation is damage of the glove material. It may get harder, softer or may swell. It will crack or tear more easily. Degradation indicates the deterioration of the glove material on contact with a named substance. Choose gloves with an excellent or good degradation rating.

51   The wearer is unlikely to notice permeation or breakthrough because inside the glove the substance is likely to be present as a vapour. The glove will not show any obvious change.

52   Once permeation has started, it continues even if the glove is no longer in contact with the substance. It only stops when the concentration of the chemical on the inside surface of the glove equals the concentration on the outer surface.

53   Protective gloves are not only subject to physical and chemical damage. Ageing, flexing and stretching, poor storage and poor maintenance all lead to deterioration of the glove and loss of protection.

54   As noted earlier, manufacturers' data are for pure chemicals, yet most products are mixtures. As a 'rule of thumb', base your glove selection on the component in the mixture/product with the shortest breakthrough time. However, the only way to be sure how a glove performs is to have it tested against the product.

Other hazards for hands

55   Are there other hazards to take into account, for example abrasion, cuts, puncture, vibration or high temperature? There are protective gloves that combine chemical protection with protection against other hazards:

- gloves marked EN388 give protection from mechanical hazards;
- gloves marked EN407 give protection from thermal hazards.

The type and duration of contact

56   Will gloves be worn for a short time, intermittently or for long periods? Generally, thicker, robust gloves offer greater protection than thinner gloves but thinner gloves offer better dexterity. For intermittent use, a series of thin 'single-use' gloves may offer adequate protection. Where thicker, reusable gloves are used intermittently, they need to be stored carefully between each use.

57   Will contact be from occasional splashes or by total immersion? Short gloves can protect against splashes but if hands are immersed (and this is unavoidable), choose a length greater than the depth of immersion.

The wearer – size and comfort

58   Wearing protective gloves can be uncomfortable, particularly when undertaking a physically demanding task and for long periods. Thick gloves restrict movement and reduce dexterity, making precise work impossible.

59   Gloves should fit the wearer. Tight gloves can make hands feel tired and lose their grip. Gloves that are too large can create folds; these can impair work and be uncomfortable – see Appendix 2 for sizing charts.

60   Employees are more likely to wear comfortable gloves. Involving them in the selection process, by giving them a reasonable choice to pick from, can sometimes promote buy-in to wearing them.

61   Hands can sweat inside gloves, making the skin over-hydrated (which can lead to dermatitis) and the gloves uncomfortable to wear. Getting staff to take glove breaks, removing gloves for a minute or so before hands get too hot and sweaty, can help air the hands. You might also supply separate cotton gloves to wear under protective gloves to help absorb sweat. They may be laundered and reused.

62   Sometimes the chemicals used in the manufacture of protective gloves can cause skin allergies in some individuals. A particular problem with single-use natural rubber latex (NRL) gloves is that proteins naturally present in the latex can also cause allergies, either through direct contact with the skin (leading to contact urticaria) or, if the gloves are powdered, by inhalation of the powder (leading to asthma).

63   If you select single-use NRL gloves, your risk assessment must have identified them as necessary, ie you identified them as the safest choice of material for a given hazardous substance and you know that those employees do not have an allergy to NRL. When provided, they must be 'low-protein and powder-free' and should carry a CE mark.

The task

64   Gloves should not hamper the task. If wet/oily objects are handled, choose gloves with a roughened/textured surface for good grip. Select gloves that balance protection with dexterity. Thick gloves are suitable for heavy-duty, less precise work. Ensure the gloves selected meet any standards required for the task, eg sterile gloves, food grade gloves. Consider whether colour is important, to show up contamination for example.

Is there anything else I need to consider?

Issue, maintenance and disposal

65   You will need to make suitable arrangements for storing, inspecting, issuing, record keeping and disposing of protective gloves.

- Make arrangements for storing an adequate stock of gloves of the right sizes and types.
- Make arrangements for the issue of gloves when they need replacement (ie based on the glove performance data, not just when they look like they have worn out or when an employee asks).
- Some glove types require maintenance – this may mean a regular inspection routine to check the state of the gloves in use or cleaning inside gloves. Follow manufacturers' instructions.
- Keep appropriate records (eg stock or maintenance issues).
- Arrange for storing and disposing of used gloves. Do they need disposal as hazardous waste?

Information, instruction and training

66   Protective gloves are only effective if they are used correctly. Employees, supervisors, managers and those involved in 'glove maintenance' need training (or refresher training) in the effective use of protective gloves. Training may appear trivial – it isn't.

67   Everyone who wears protective gloves needs to know:

- what gloves to wear and when to wear them;
- how to look after them;
- how to put them on and take them off without contaminating the skin;
- the limitations of gloves as a control measure;
- how to dispose of them safely.

68   Refresher training will be particularly important for people who do not have to wear protective gloves very often, or are likely to use them only for emergency purposes such as dealing with spillages.

69   It is advisable to keep records of training details.

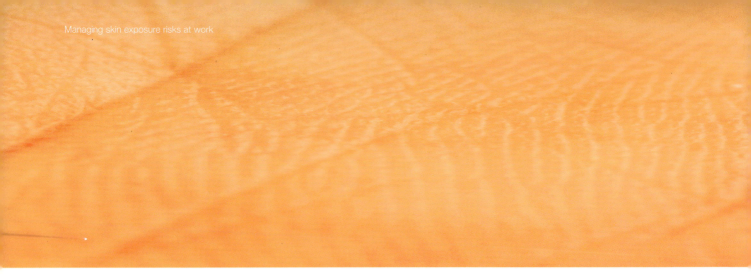

Case study: Cleaner exposed to detergents

A part-time cleaner developed severe dermatitis as a result of exposure to detergents she used at work. She sued her employer. In defence, her employer told the court that she had been supplied with rubber gloves.

On investigation, it was found that she had been supplied with gloves but was unaware of, and had not been told about, the risk of dermatitis from exposure to detergents.

To make matters worse, she had not been instructed in the steps she needed to take to protect herself. The cleaner won the case and was awarded substantial damages.

Costs

70   Generally, single-use gloves are fairly inexpensive, common reusable gloves can cost a few pounds a pair and specialist gloves can be tens of pounds a pair. The factors that influence the costs depend on the buyer's purchasing power and some are shown below:

- the size of a specific order;
- the likelihood of repeat orders;
- the size of the purchasing body.

71   When you assess the cost of implementing a protective glove programme, you will need to consider:

- initial purchase and replacement;
- any costs associated with issue, storage and disposal;
- any costs associated with training.

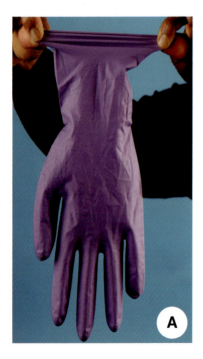
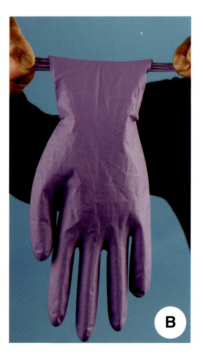
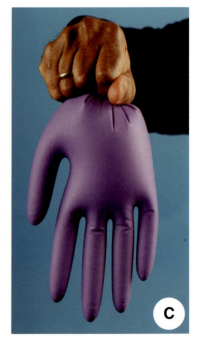

A simple method for detecting fine holes in a glove. A - stretch the cuff of the glove, trapping a small amount of air inside. B - fold the cuff over several times to compress the air. C - if the glove is hole-free, it should remain inflated like this.

Protection with good skin care

72 Skin care will help to protect the skin by reducing the effects of exposure.

- Accidental contamination should be washed away promptly.
- Encourage employees to wash areas of skin that may have been exposed to hazardous substances at breaks and after work. They should wash the skin with warm water and dry thoroughly, preferably with a clean, dry, soft towel.
- Provide clean washing facilities as near as possible to the area of work. Provide the least aggressive cleaning products that will do the job and never allow solvents or very abrasive products to be used for skin cleaning.
- Pre-work creams can be applied before starting work or on returning from a break.
- After-work creams should be used to replace the natural oils that the skin can lose when washed or when it comes into contact with detergents.

Choosing and using skin care products

73 Skin care products are designed to help maintain a stable and adequately hydrated barrier layer so the skin remains in good condition and retains its protective role.

Pre-work creams

74 These are designed for application at the start of work, after breaks etc, and there are several types.

- Vanishing creams trap contaminants such as resins and dyes, which can then be washed off the skin. They may contain refined mineral oil, petrolatum, lanolin, emulsifiers, preservatives and fragrances.
- Water-resistant creams form a film over the skin surface that repels water-based chemicals such as acids and alkalis. They can contain silicones, beeswax, stearates, preservatives, fragrances and synthetic tanning agents. Water-resistant creams tend to feel greasy.
- Oil/organic solvent-resistant creams are designed to repel oils, tars and organic solvents. They may contain glycerine, preservatives and fragrances. These creams can come off through sweating.
- Other types of pre-work cream react chemically with the contaminant to make it less harmful, for example by reacting with acids to make them less acidic, or trapping an allergen such as nickel.

75 Choose creams that have the best repellant properties for the substances in your workplace.

76 Sometimes pre-work creams are known as 'barrier creams' but this is something of a misnomer and may lull users into a false sense of security. Pre-work creams do not function as protective gloves and employees should not use them in their place. Some pre-work creams appear to provide some protection against the substances for which they were designed. However, others seem to give far less protection in practice than their formulations suggest. They do not a form a barrier in the same way that personal protective equipment (PPE) does because:

- workers may not apply them properly, leaving part of their skin unprotected;
- there is no information available on the rate of penetration of substances through pre-work creams;
- they may be removed while working, without workers noticing.

77 Pre-work creams can play a role in an overall skin care programme. They will help remove dirt during washing, so milder cleansing agents can be used.

Case study: Pre-work creams, moisturisers and gloves

Pete was a motor mechanic who loved his job. He was always getting oil, grease and petrol on his hands from handling dirty parts and equipment. Pete often used his bare hands to remove parts soaking in a bucket of solvent. He didn't use the gloves he was given because he thought they made the work hard.

Pete used a strong, abrasive cleaner to get the dirt off whenever he washed his hands. Pete ended up with dermatitis and had to have a number of weeks off, to let his hands heal. When he came back to work a number of changes had been introduced. Pete now also does his bit and his dermatitis has not come back.

- A cleaning station is now used to degrease parts.
- Pete persevered with using gloves for tasks where he couldn't avoid contact with hazardous materials, and he gradually got used to them.
- Pre-work creams are used. They make it easier to remove dirt when washing, so the abrasive hand cleaner has been replaced with a milder one.
- Moisturisers are supplied and used.
- Skin checks are carried out.

Skin cleansers

78 These remove contaminants from the skin, but they can also damage it. A suitable cleanser will remove most of a particular contaminant without causing unacceptable damage to the skin. Some products may contain components intended to moisturise the skin, and counteract the damaging effects of surface-active agents (surfactants), which are present in most skin cleansers. There are three main components of skin cleansers:

- Surfactants (eg soap) wetten and suspend dirt in water, which is then removed by washing. Washing with water alone may spread contaminants around the skin, rather than remove them. The skin may be damaged by surfactants. There are different types of surfactants in skin cleansers that vary in their skin compatibility. The pH of a cleanser (a measure of its acidity or alkalinity) is not usually a reliable guide to its tolerance by the skin.
- Scrubbing agents (heavy-duty cleansers) mechanically remove contaminants by their abrasive action. They may also be designed to attract loosened particles onto their surfaces. Sand, the original scrubbing agent, was very aggressive. Avoid very abrasive products; milder abrasives such as wood flours and plastics are preferred. Another alternative is walnut shell powder.
- Organic solvents are present in certain cleansers to dissolve contaminants such as paint. All organic solvents can remove the natural fat in the skin to some degree. Milder solvents such as alkanes and acetates are preferred.

79 You should use the least aggressive cleanser that will do the job.

Moisturisers

80 Whether a cream, lotion or ointment, these are all moisturisers. They are also known as 'emollients' or skin conditioners. Their purpose is to help replace moisture and temporarily restore the barrier effect of the skin. This allows the moisture in the barrier layer to be restored by natural processes within the body. They need to be applied at least once a day, preferably more frequently, and ideally each time the hands are washed and dried.

81 The basic components of after-work creams are water, oils and emulsifiers. Water is sometimes the main component. The most common oils are refined mineral oil, petrolatum and lanolin; these coat the skin and reduce the amount of water lost by evaporation. After-work creams may also include preservatives, fragrances and other ingredients.

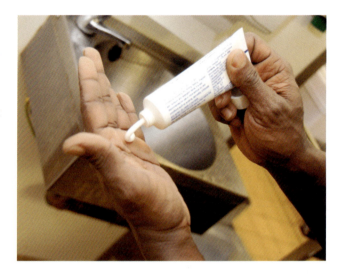

One of a number of dispenser types for moisturiser. Dispensers are preferred to tubs to reduce the likelihood of cross contamination.

Choosing skin care products

82 When choosing skin care products, bear in mind the following points.

- The choice of products should be appropriate to the hazards in your workplace and suitable for each employee. Ask suppliers for help.
- Will the product do the job? Is there evidence to support claims?
- Is a full list of ingredients provided? Can any cause dermatitis?
- Products should be placed in appropriate places, eg by sinks, not too far from work areas.
- Is educational support for the product available, eg leaflets or videos?
- Inform and instruct employees on their use.
- Ask suppliers to help you select a suitable skin care product.
- Dispensing systems need to be easy to use and replenish – keep a stock.

83 Certain ingredients of skin care products are known to be skin sensitisers. If you suspect a worker has developed an allergy to a skin care product, it can only be confirmed by specific skin tests known as 'patch tests'. These should only be carried out under the supervision of a skin specialist, preferably a dermatologist. In the first instance, workers may be referred to their GP, or company occupational health nurse or doctor if there is one.

Check for early signs of skin disease

84   When employees are exposed to hazardous substances, employers need to ensure that, where appropriate, employees are under suitable health surveillance. The following paragraphs refer to carrying out health surveillance for 'local effects' following skin exposure to hazardous substances, ie straightforward visual checks of employees' skin.

85   To find out if it is appropriate to carry out health surveillance for 'systemic effects', or for further information on whether skin checks are appropriate, the first thing to do is to look at HSE guidance relevant to your business. You can find information on this in HSE's more detailed guidance on health surveillance.[5]

Why should skin checks be carried out?

86   Skin checks are a crucial part of managing skin disease at work.

- Regular skin checks will help to identify the early stages of dermatitis or other skin effects caused by skin exposure.
- The earlier that health effects are recognised and treated, the more likely it is that the sufferer will make a full recovery.
- Checks can also show whether an adequate standard of control is being maintained. They may give an early indication of lapses in control and the need for a reassessment of the control strategy.

Case study: Hairdressing

Maureen had been a hairdresser for many years and eventually owned her own salon. When she returned to work after having a family she spotted a rash on the back of her hands. She initially ignored it. However, her hands swelled up and starting cracking and the rash spread all over her body. It became infected. Wet work had damaged Maureen's skin, leaving it vulnerable.

She subsequently developed an allergy to an ingredient in a hair product. She used steroid creams prescribed by her doctor to treat it, but work was becoming a struggle. Her home life suffered too. Simple tasks such as washing dishes or peeling potatoes, even bathing the children, caused her immense pain.

This could have been avoided if the right preventative measures had been followed:

- wearing suitable gloves for washing clients' hair and using chemicals;
- if products got on her hands, rinsing them, then drying them thoroughly;
- using a moisturiser regularly;
- seeing her doctor earlier.

Who should carry out skin checks?

87   Employers using substances with a potential to cause skin disease should conduct regular skin checks. Checks for skin diseases can be as simple as conducting regular visual inspection of the potentially exposed areas of workers' skin. A 'responsible person' should carry out skin checks but employees should be encouraged to check their own skin and to report any problems promptly. You need to safeguard the confidentiality of such reports.

88   The role of a responsible person is to:

- assess the condition of a new employee's skin before, or as soon as possible after, they start work;
- periodically check the skin of employees' hands and forearms for the early signs of skin disease;
- keep secure health records of these checks;
- tell the employer the outcome of these checks, for any remedial action; and
- advise the employer when to seek expert help on any skin disease outbreak, and for restoring control of exposure.

89   A 'responsible person' can be an employee provided with suitable training. They should know:

- the substances in their workplace that can cause skin disease;
- the types of skin diseases they can cause;
- what the early signs of those diseases look like;
- how exposure happens through handling, use, maintenance etc;
- what controls are in place and the consequences of any shortcomings;
- what action to take on finding a problem. This includes:
  - reporting to the employer on the disease and exposure controls;
  - advising the affected employee(s) to see their GP;
  - keeping records of observations;
  - keeping records secure.

Summary

90   Manage the work in your workplace to prevent skin and systemic disease. Ask yourself whether you have to use a hazardous substance or whether you can use a safer alternative. If you have to use hazardous substances then you should ensure suitable controls are in place to avoid or reduce exposure. If exposure is unavoidable, you will also need to protect workers' skin (through PPE and skin care).

91   Remember that worker behaviour is critical in determining the effectiveness of control measures. Studies have shown that skin exposure is often increased by poor work practices. Engineering controls and PPE programmes are unlikely to be fully effective unless they are supported by appropriate levels of management. It is important to regularly inform, instruct and train employees about the risks to health from skin exposure and the precautions needed to prevent disease.

92   You need to check your controls, check for skin disease and, where appropriate, introduce health surveillance for systemic diseases and investigate any incidents. Make sure any employees with work-related health problems receive medical treatment.

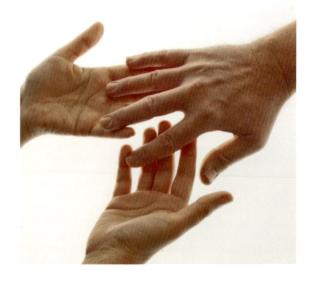

Health surveillance for 'local effects' can be as simple as visual checks of employees' skin.

Avoid	Protect	Check
Examples of ways to avoid contact	**Examples of ways to protect skin**	**Reasons for skin checks**
■ Substitute a more hazardous material with a safer alternative. ■ Automate the process. ■ Enclose the process as much as possible. ■ Use mechanical handling. ■ Use equipment for handling. ■ Don't use the hands as tools. ■ Use a safe working distance.	■ Tell workers how to look after their skin. ■ Remind them to wash any contamination from their skin promptly. ■ Tell them about the importance of thorough drying after washing. ■ Provide soft cotton or paper towels. ■ Supply moisturising pre-work and after-work creams. ■ Provide appropriate protective clothing/gloves. ■ Make sure gloves are made of suitable material. ■ Select gloves that are the right size and right for the task to be done. ■ Use and store gloves correctly. ■ Replace gloves when necessary. ■ Provide training for safe glove removal.	■ Regular skin checks can spot the early stages of dermatitis. ■ Early detection can prevent more serious dermatitis from developing. ■ Steps can be taken to start treating the condition. ■ Checks can help indicate a possible lapse in your preventative measures and the need to reassess the situation.

Appendix 1 What does the relevant law say?

1   The Health and Safety at Work etc Act 1974 (the HSW Act)[6] and several sets of regulations are most relevant to the control of risks to health which arise from skin exposure to hazardous substances at work. These regulations are:

- the Control of Substances Hazardous to Health Regulations 2002 (as amended) (COSHH);[7]
- the Management of Health and Safety at Work Regulations 1999;[8]
- the Chemical (Hazard Information and Packaging for Supply) Regulations 1994 (CHIP);[4]
- the Personal Protective Equipment at Work Regulations 1992.[9,10]

HSW Act

2   The HSW Act is an umbrella Act concerned with securing the health, safety and welfare of people at work, and with protecting those who are not at work from the risks to their health and safety from work activities. An employer's main duties with respect to skin exposure are to:

- prevent or adequately control exposure to substances that cause damage to the health of employees and others (eg contractors or visitors) affected by work activities under their control;
- ensure hazardous substances are used safely;
- ensure safe systems of work are in place and followed;
- ensure equipment and tools are safe and maintained;
- provide free personal protective clothing or equipment where it is necessary;
- provide adequate welfare facilities, including skin care products;
- provide health surveillance as appropriate;
- give employees information, instruction, training and supervision;
- appoint a competent person(s) to assist with health and safety responsibilities;
- consult employees or their safety representative;
- set up emergency procedures;
- provide adequate first-aid facilities;
- ensure appropriate safety signs are provided and maintained;
- report diseases to the appropriate health and safety enforcing authority (eg HSE).

3   Employees have a legal duty to co-operate with their employer by correctly using the safe systems of work provided, in particular to:

- take reasonable care for their own health and safety and that of others who may be affected by what they do or do not do;
- co-operate with the employer on health and safety;
- correctly use work items provided by the employer, including personal protective equipment;
- use all safe systems of work in accordance with training or instructions;
- not interfere with or misuse anything provided for health, safety or welfare.

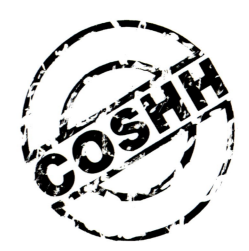

COSHH

4   COSHH provides a legal framework to protect people against health risks from hazardous substances used at work. It applies wherever there is a risk at work of health effects from skin exposure to hazardous substances. COSHH requires employers to:

- assess the risk from hazardous substances and wet work;
- prevent or adequately control the risk with control measures;
- record the findings of the assessment for five or more employees;
- maintain and monitor the effectiveness of controls in place;
- in some situations to carry out air monitoring and health surveillance;
- inform, instruct and train the workforce about the risks of exposure to substances hazardous to health and the precautions that should be taken.

CHIP

5   CHIP requires suppliers to identify the hazards of the chemicals they supply, to give the hazard information to their customers and to package their chemicals appropriately. CHIP applies to most chemicals but not all. Some chemicals, such as cosmetics and medicines, are outside the scope and have their own specific laws.

6   All over the world, there are different laws on how to identify the hazardous properties of chemicals. The UK is committed to the development of a global scheme for the classification and labelling of chemicals through the UN. This long-term project will require new law (EU and UK) to be put in place. When this happens, the CHIP Regulations will be repealed in full in the UK (anticipated to be June 2015).

7   It may be necessary to amend CHIP and its supporting guidance as the transitional period progresses and the new Regulations begin to apply the new GHS (Globally Harmonised System) regime. To find out more about GHS, visit the HSE web pages at www.hse.gov.uk/ghs.

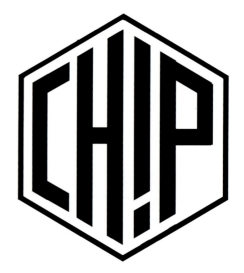

Personal Protective Equipment at Work Regulations 1992

8   These Regulations concern the design, construction, testing and certification of protective clothing and other types of PPE. They require PPE to be cleaned, maintained, used and stored properly.

Appendix 2 Glove sizes - measuring your hand

Length

Measure from the bottom edge of your palm to the tip of your middle finger to determine your 'finger length' size.

EU sizes		US sizes		
160 mm	EU - 6	6 5/16 inches	XS	
171 mm	EU - 7	6 3/4 inches	S	
182 mm	EU - 8	7 3/16 inches	M	
192 mm	EU - 9	7 9/16 inches	L	
204 mm	EU - 10	8 1/16 inches	XL	
215 plus mm	EU - 11	8 7/16 plus inches	XXL	

Width

Wrap a measuring tape around your dominant hand just below your knuckles, excluding your thumb, and make a fist. This measurement is your 'hand width' glove size.

EU sizes		US sizes		
152-178 mm	EU - 6	6-7 inches	XS	
178-203 mm	EU - 7	7-8 inches	S	
203-229 mm	EU - 8	8-9 inches	M	
229-254 mm	EU - 9	9-10 inches	L	
254-279 mm	EU - 10	10-11 inches	XL	
279 plus mm	EU - 11	11 plus inches	XXL	

Appendix 3 Memory aid for selecting protective gloves

Company:	Reference:
Department:	**Date:**
Contact:	**Number of workers:**

Description of task:

<table>
<tr><td colspan="5" align="center">Substance handled:</td></tr>
<tr><td colspan="5">☐ Wet work   ☐ Hazardous substances</td></tr>
<tr>
<td>Substance</td>
<td>Form
(solid, liquid,
gas etc)</td>
<td>Concentration</td>
<td>Temperature
(during use)</td>
<td>Label or Material
Safety Data Sheet
(MSDS) attached?</td>
</tr>
<tr><td></td><td></td><td></td><td></td><td></td></tr>
<tr><td></td><td></td><td></td><td></td><td></td></tr>
<tr><td></td><td></td><td></td><td></td><td></td></tr>
<tr><td></td><td></td><td></td><td></td><td></td></tr>
<tr><td></td><td></td><td></td><td></td><td></td></tr>
</table>

Other hazards present:

Mechanical:

☐ Snag   ☐ Puncture   ☐ Abrasion   ☐ Cut   ☐ Tear

Thermal:

☐ Heat   ☐ Cold   ☐ Hot splashes   ☐ Hot sparks ☐

Biological:

☐ Infectious material (bacteria, viruses etc)   ☐ Body fluids (blood, urine etc)

Other (eg antistatic needed, radiation protection needed):

Type and duration of contact:

Type of contact:

☐ Accidental splash   ☐ Direct contact   ☐ Immersion (note depth)   ☐ Deposition

Duration of contact:

☐ Occasional contact (note maximum contact time)

☐ Continual contact (note maximum contact time)

Wearer requirements:

Sizes required:

Inner gloves required:

Length of arm to be protected:

Any known skin allergies or other considerations:

Task requirements:

Grip requirements:

☐ Dry grip   ☐ Wet grip   ☐ Oily

Dexterity requirements:

☐ Precision   ☐ Some dexterity   ☐ Optimum protection, dexterity less important

Colour requirements (eg to show up contamination):

Special requirements (eg sterile, food grade):

References

1   Kintz, P, Tracqui, A, and Mangin P 'Accidental death caused by the absorption of 2,4-dichlorophenol through the skin' *Arch Toxicol* **66**, 298-299 (1992)

2   Ohi, G and Wegman DH 'Transcutaneous Ethylene Glycol Monomethyl Ether Poisoning in the Work Setting' *J Occup Med* **20**, 675-76 (1978)

3   *EH40/2005 Workplace exposure limits: Containing the list of workplace exposure limits for use with the Control of Substances Hazardous to Health Regulations 2002 (as amended)* Environmental Hygiene Guidance Note EH40 HSE Books 2005 ISBN 978 0 7176 2977 0

4   *CHIP for everyone* HSG228 HSE Books 2002 ISBN 978 0 7176 2370 9

5   *Understanding health surveillance at work: An introduction for employers* Leaflet INDG304 HSE Books 1999 (single copy free or priced packs of 15 ISBN 978 0 7176 1712 8) www.hse.gov.uk/pubns/indg304.pdf

6   *Health and Safety at Work etc Act 1974 (c.37)* The Stationery Office 1974 ISBN 978 0 10 543774 1

7   *Control of substances hazardous to health (Fifth edition). The Control of Substances Hazardous to Health Regulations 2002 (as amended). Approved Code of Practice and guidance* L5 (Fifth edition) HSE Books 2005 ISBN 978 0 7176 2981 7

8   *Management of health and safety at work. Management of Health and Safety at Work Regulations 1999. Approved Code of Practice and guidance* L21 (Second edition) HSE Books 2000 ISBN 978 0 7176 2488 1

9   *Personal protective equipment at work (Second edition). Personal Protective Equipment at Work Regulations 1992 (as amended). Guidance on Regulations* L25 (Second edition) HSE Books 2005 ISBN 978 0 7176 6139 8

10   *A short guide to the Personal Protective Equipment at Work Regulations 1992* Leaflet INDG174(rev1) HSE Books 2005 (single copy free or priced packs of 15 ISBN 978 0 7176 6141 1) www.hse.gov.uk/pubns/indg174.pdf

Further reading

Five steps to risk assessment Leaflet INDG163(rev2)
HSE Books 2006 (single copy free or priced packs of 10
ISBN 978 0 7176 6189 3)
www.hse.gov.uk/pubns/indg163.pdf

*A guide to the Reporting of Injuries, Diseases and
Dangerous Occurrences Regulations 1995* L73 (Third
edition) HSE Books 2008 ISBN 978 0 7176 6290 6

*PUWER 1998: Provision and Use of Work Equipment
Regulations 1998: Open learning guidance* HSE Books
2008 ISBN 978 0 7176 6285 2

*Controlling skin exposure to chemicals and wet-work:
A practical book* RMS Publishing 2008
ISBN 978 1 906674 00 7

COSHH essentials: www.coshh-essentials.org.uk

HSE's Skin at work website: www.hse.gov.uk/skin

Further information

HSE priced and free publications are available by mail order from HSE Books, PO Box 1999, Sudbury, Suffolk CO10 2WA Tel: 01787 881165 Fax: 01787 313995 Website: www.hsebooks.co.uk (HSE priced publications are also available from bookshops and free leaflets can be downloaded from HSE's website: www.hse.gov.uk.)

For information about health and safety ring HSE's Infoline Tel: 0845 345 0055 Fax: 0845 408 9566 Textphone: 0845 408 9577 e-mail: hse.infoline@natbrit.com or write to HSE Information Services, Caerphilly Business Park, Caerphilly CF83 3GG.

The Stationery Office publications are available from The Stationery Office, PO Box 29, Norwich NR3 1GN Tel: 0870 600 5522 Fax: 0870 600 5533 e-mail: customer.services@tso.co.uk Website: www.tso.co.uk (They are also available from bookshops.) Statutory Instruments can be viewed free of charge at www.opsi.gov.uk.

Training courses

Those wishing to improve their knowledge and skills can obtain qualifications such as:

British Occupational Hygiene Society (BOHS) P801: Control of dermal exposure at work.

BOHS can also give advice on training courses. For more information you can contact them at:

BOHS, 5/6 Melbourne Business Court
Millennium Way
Pride Park
Derby
DE24 8LZ

Tel: 01332 298101
Fax: 01332 298099
e-mail: admin@bohs.org
website: www.bohs.org

Printed and published by the Health and Safety Executive
C75   01/09